I0447546

Weight Loss Diets

Easy tips for loss weight and long term results

Kate Garcia

CONTENTS

INTRODUCTION

Diet...The notion that appears more and more every day. Today, more and more people struggle with being overweight and bad welfare. We usually start fighting our extra weight with diets, but that is a common mistake that normally doesn't bring real results. There is almost no man who hasn't faced and tried a diet in his life. Every spring offers different diets; better, more efficient.

I first came in contact with a diet in my early teenage years. I didn't have too much weight, but I wasn't happy with my body. I always read different magazines and newspapers with tips on how to reach a better body, how to get rid of cellulite, how to get nicely toned legs, what to eat to feel better, to have better hair, hard nails, and much more. All promised miraculous results.

But, in my case, the result was completely opposite. Pants from last year were too tight, and my dress size kept going up. There was even more visible cellulite. The less I ate,

the worse the results and my mood became.

All those diets have lead me to anemia and stomach pains when eating certain foods. And so I ended up in a vicious circle from which I didn't see an exit, despite all the tips in magazines, newspapers, and on the Internet that I've read. All of them want to help, give tips, but in the end, you're alone, dissatisfied with yourself.

Often, there is nothing else left but being dissatisfied with yourself. Improper diet can lead to many serious situations and diseases like cardiovascular diseases, cholesterol, high blood pressure, cancer, etc.

More than two thirds of people die as a result of non-communicable chronic diseases. Poor nutrition and irregular lifestyle has a big role in that. But good news follows. We can prevent the majority of chronic diseases like obesity, cancer, cardiovascular diseases, and diabetes with a healthy lifestyle. That means healthy diet and exercise.

WHAT IS DIET

Diet means balanced way of eating. It means an individual tries to eat the most healthy and varied food.

Diet doesn't mean that we don't eat. Often, my clients tell me that if they want to lose some weight, they don't eat for a few days and lose a few kilograms. Some say it's best to sew your mouth together.

And then what? In a week, two weeks, and if you're patient, in one month, but the maximum of one month, you return to the same, if not worse, position you were in before. In best case, you gain back all the kg you lost. In a worst case, you gain an extra 10 kilograms. In even worse case, you could have attracted a disease.

So it really should not be that easy to accept the tips that media or friends give us! It is your body, your health! I find it terrible when I hear people who come in my office, and tell, with pride, what way they lost their weight. When I measure them on analyzer of body composition, they are shocked. They can't believe that their ratio between fat and muscles is completely wrong.

The Main Reason for Malaise and Being Overweight

Our health is largely dependent on the diet of our cells. That is most noticeable on your skin and nails. Different creams relieve our outer problems, but they don't eliminate the causes. Skin problems are often the response of prolonged lack of nutrients.

As long as there's not that many injured or badly fed cells, we don't notice that. When there's a large number of injured cells, the irregularities of the skin are often visible and disturbing. Often, just a little change of diet is enough to improve skin health. Beauty and youthful appearance are very important in today's social value. That's the reason more and more people are aware of the importance of a balanced diet. Despite the rapid pace of life, that's not a problem, as healthy, tasty fast food is widely available on the market.

Fast Pace of Life

How many times did you think today, "I'm in a hurry, fast, fast!"? Once, five times, ten times?

Our fast pace of life has completely backed us into a corner. Despite the knowledge and technological progress, we have become slaves. Fast pace of life dictates that we should not take much care of our own and basic well-being: health.

Health comes from food, as peppers, potatoes, and salad get displaced into molecules in our digestive system. Those molecules become a part of us. Really, pepper turns into us. Body needs building blocks, like proteins, minerals, and vitamins. If we don't give it the requested nutrients, it adapts to the situation. That adaptation is not eternal and omnipotent.

Over time, our body fails; the stamina leaves us. We are tired all the time, in a bad mood, depressed. Soon, we need unusually large amounts of sleep so we relax to some extent. If we don't do anything to change the situation, disease is imminent.

We don't take any time – even to eat. In the "lack of" time, we eschew to unhealthy fast food and eat less and less fresh fruit and vegetables. Industrially pre-prepared food often comes from animal sources and has hidden preservatives, sugar, fat, and salt.

It is heat treated and contains food additives, food coloring, and aromas, which allow longer freshness and shelf life. Food like that doesn't provide an adequate supply of vitamins and minerals to the body, which are essential for the maintenance of healthy and general welfare.

The content of nutrients in food prepared in such way is small. It also contains many harmful substances, which, with years of insufficient nutrition, accumulate in our bodies. That food is, on the other hand, very energy-rich, which only worsens the situation, because we eat too much energy, which is stored in the form of fat.

22 million of children are overweight – that number is estimated to increase by 1.3 million until the year of 2010. Obesity is often not treated as a serious problem – the majority of people argue that obesity concerned others more than ourselves. Denial of the problem doesn't change the fact that obesity often leads to serious diseases of the cardiovascular system and diabetes.

Before we decide on any diet, we must first ask ourselves:

1. Is my frustration really related to my weight?

I was not overweight. Based on my height, I had just the right weight. That means that my frustration was a result of something else. I needed confirmation from others. Of course, I didn't realize that at the given moment. Things like that often happen in adolescents, who feel the lack of attention from their parents. However, even older people are not an exception.

2.   How many kilograms do I want to lose or what do I want to reach?

Like I mentioned before, I wasn't overweight, but I had some extra body fat on some parts of my body – on the parts we normally don't want to have any fat. I suggest to everyone that before you pick a diet, you get an assessment of body composition (it can be made by a wellness coach – some even do it for free). That way, you can track your progress and see if you're actually losing fat or muscle mass. Many people give too much attention to weight, and too little to the composition of their body. It is healthier to have less fat and more muscle mass. Muscle mass is denser than fat, so its volume is less. Therefore, the right way to track our progress is by dress size and measurements rather than weight.

3.   Set realistic goals

You want to lose 30 kilograms. You plan to lose 10 of those in the first week. Is it possible? Maybe, but not in a healthy and realistic way. It's best to take small steps.

4. Take pictures and measure your sizes (e.g., Chest, waist, hips). Measure yourself once a week – if possible, at the same time of the day and the same day of the week (e.g., on Friday at 9am).

WHY DON'T DIETS WORK?

One of the very serious diseases of the Western world is obesity. Almost 2/3 of people in America are overweight. Obesity has become a serious problem, as it can lead to many serious conditions like cardiovascular diseases, diabetes, etc. It is very worrying that more and more children suffer from obesity. On the other hand, there's a new slimming diet that promises lasting wonders in just a few days, almost every day. And so, sometimes it's recommended to eat just meat and other animal food sources, and other times to count points or calories. And then someone discovers that his/her diet is the best. You won't like this information, but only 2% of those who lose weight permanently get rid of unwanted kilograms! So why is it like that? Why don't the slimming diets work?

- First reason is based on the fact that people stick to the diet for a certain time, but then return to their old way of eating. But their old ways actually lead to the reason they started the diet in the first place! If you continue living a certain lifestyle that you were living before the diet, the result can't be different than it was before – extra kilograms.

-They are concerned only with weight loss instead of focusing on losing the body fat percentage.

General weight loss gets rid of a lot of muscle mass, which is actually the main component of fat burning.

Weight loss is too fast, which leads to the body's natural defence mechanism kicking in, which causes the maximum preservation of fat.

The real purpose of weight reduction is getting rid of body fat while retaining all the muscle mass and water. None of the current weight loss programs attempt to distinguish between the three weight components. Some programs are designed to partially dehydrate the participants to show certain 'success'. Any high school wrestler or judoist can tell you how to lose 2.5 liters of water in two days – with the cessation of drinking, sitting in sauna, taking diuretic pills, or ingesting diuretic foods like melon or real coffee. But such tactics stimulate the body to produce even more of the anti-diuretic hormone, which leads to retention of every water drop once you start drinking normally again. We know that dehydration destroys health and sports performance.

Another big problem of commercial diets is the greater stimulation of the body to accumulate fat after you start dieting. As a result of human desire of fast results, the diets have a low daily calorie allowance (800 – 1.200 kcal). Under eating to that point causes fast loss of muscle mass. The body has a built-in natural defence mechanism, which recognizes the fat loss as an attack on its energy reserve, so it immediately initiates various defence operations. Two of those operations especially destroy your efforts to get rid of fat. Firstly, your body increases the amount and activity of the enzyme lipoprotein lipase, the main enzyme used to collect and store fat. Then your metabolic rate is slowed, which further reduces your ability to burn fat.

How to eat to maintain a healthy body weight and health

Breakfast

Like I mentioned before, diet means a healthy way of eating. The first important thing is that we should never skip breakfast. Breakfast is the most important meal of the day, but 70% of people skip it. Many studies were done about this topic. They all show that proverbs such as "After the breakfast the day shows" or "Eat breakfast like a king, and dine like a beggar," hold some truth. Breakfast is a meal that should be eaten as soon as possible after we wake up, not when we come to work like many people do.

Many times, when I talk to my customers, I like to compare our bodies with cars. Imagine that you bought the car of your dreams. You paid more than $80,100 for it. You go on a long drive. When will you fill its tank? In the beginning, or will you drive 10 km and only then give fuel to it? Every time you stop at the gas station, what time of fuel do you choose? Cheapest? Best?

When it's time to change its oil, which one do you choose? The cheapest one? When the yellow or red light shines on the dashboard, do you ignore it and drive on or go to the closest mechanic?

And when it comes to our body, which has parts that are not that easy to replace – we don't care? In the morning, we drink a cup of coffee on an empty stomach, light a cigarette, go to work, where we are followed by stress and other different physical and mental troubles. *And* then in 20 – 30 years, we ask ourselves, why does this happen to me? Why do I have this disease? Or we console ourselves that this is hereditary, because our mom or grandmother had it. The truth is, 30% of diseases are hereditary, and the other 70% depend on us – on our diet and activity. We inherit only the same habits. Shopping and eating habits.

Are you maybe one of those people who do eat breakfast every day, but it consists of simple carbohydrates like white bread, cocoa, croissants, cereals,...

So, it is not only important to have breakfast, but to have a right one, too. And this is the point where trouble begins if you don't have enough knowledge. Today, it's hard to consume the sufficient amount of nutrients our body needs. Because we don't have enough knowledge, or someone who has enough knowledge, this is even harder. I don't mean knowledge from magazines and newspapers, which are full of tips that are often taken from the wrong sources.

So, how should a healthy breakfast look like? We need to eat all the nutrients our body needs (carbohydrates, proteins, fats, vitamins, and minerals). Carbohydrates should be complex, which means eating wholegrain bread or unprocessed cereal (Muesli). You can find proteins in eggs, dairy products,... besides that, you have to pick a fruit and vegetables, which provide vitamins and minerals. Fastest and easiest way to eat the necessary nutrients is to consume a meal replacement product, but choose one that a scientist developed.

The Meals during the Day

During the day, have well-spaced healthy meals. That means you should eat every 3 to 4 hours. Not large quantities but small meals. That can be fruit, yoghurt, soy yoghurt, and protein bars with few calories and no added sugar. It can also be sandwich on whole wheat bread, nuts,... Beware of the quantity!

Avoid restaurants that offer fast food. It's not good to have a cheat meal often, as that can lead to developing a habit. Studies show that those who eat fast food at least twice a week gain 10 kg more than other people.

Eating in restaurants is a routine for many people, who spend many hours at work, but it should be noted, that eating "outside" has a very significant impact on healthy eating and body weight. Trying to condone the eating in restaurants with a "promise" to eat healthy at home the next day simply doesn't work! Every meal should start with a portion of vegetables, a salad or vegetable soup. Order a food that allows you to save on some calories – ask the chef to serve the sauce on the side. Choose a cooked, not fried, fish with a salad instead of chips and fresh fruit instead of a dessert.

Choose a menu that contains fish and lots of vegetables. Reduce your carbohydrates and increase the protein. If you're still hungry, don't order a dessert. Instead offer another portion of protein rich food.

Make the necessary changes of your eating habits and remember that this change (as a part of healthy and balanced lifestyle) is a long process and can't be done from today to tomorrow. When you choose food, do it in the wider perspective of your ideas about diet and not according to the criteria of "good" and "bad" food.

Water

It's necessary to drink enough plain water for health. The World Health Organization recommends that we drink a litre of water for every 25 kilograms of our body weight. When I first heard about this information, I started drinking flavoured water. Only later, when I got more information, I noticed that I wasn't seeing any results. Flavoured waters are hidden calories. We think that we're drinking water, but we're actually drinking colourless juice. For long term results, you have to eliminate soda and other fizzy drinks from your diet. Get used to drinking natural juices. It's even better if you make them yourself from different fruits and vegetables. At the beginning, it may not be tasty or easy. You have to remember that you're doing it for your body and the goals you wrote down at the beginning. Each new habit requires time to get used to. You have to insist! All valuable things are valuable, because not everyone can reach them! Let this be the time when you insist and reach your goal. It's worth the effort. Believe me, I, too, went over it. It's not just about a nice figure. It's much more – figure is just one of visible consequences. It's about health, energy, good mood, vitality,... It's about the fact that until now, you didn't have enough energy for all your tasks but now, some is left to do other things. All of a sudden, you have the will for sport activities, which you didn't like until now.

Dinner

I tried not to eat after a certain time. When I was alone, I somehow managed, but when I was at home with my parents, I tried but I wasn't successful. When I saw someone else eating, I gave up and joined them. I'm a person who loves to eat. I can't stand the hunger and watching people eat when I'm hungry.

For many people, dinner is the most important meal of the day, as it's the only time when they spend some time with the family. Dinner shouldn't be abundant and should be based on protein and vegetables. Don't eat too late. I recommend that you eat at least 2 to 3 hours before bed. I don't suggest that you skip the meal – instead, get used to choosing and preparing a healthy dinner.

I don't know if you were ever one of those people who didn't want to eat dinner so as not to gain weight, but then woke up in the middle of the night feeling hungry. Horrible feeling. You get up and walk to the fridge with a wish to eat something small and non-fattening. But, when you get to the fridge, the brain and reasoning turn off. The hand reaches for the sweetest (MOST fattening) food and automatically puts it in the mouth without any control. When your reasoning is back, the plate is empty. You realize that you ate a lot and start feeling awful. You're angry with yourself. Once again, you're in a vicious circle...

So don't skip meals and the feelings will no longer appear. Our body needs some nutrients in the evening, so it can properly renew.

Exercise

I never liked exercise. In primary and high school, gym was a mandatory subject, but later, my only exercise was the walk to college and back home. To work and home. Ever since I decided to eat healthy, I also got the will to run, go to the gym. But don't think that I don't ever eat a pizza, ice cream, or desserts. I do, but not every day... For some time now, I've been going to the gym for an hour when I have a lunch break at work. Last year, I attended a charity run for the first time. I ran 9 kilometres and my pace was great (not only in my opinion).

When you become more active, you can eat more things that you like, but you'll nevertheless gain fat. Therefore, just take a hike! You'll notice that after a few weeks of eating healthy and exercising, you won't even think about some foods that you constantly think about right now.

If running seems boring, you can try some other sports that also effect fat burning such as swimming, table tennis or biking. It's important that you try out different sport activities, because that is the only way to find the one that is written on your skin. Don't forget that the fact is that cardio does help you lose weight, but your body won't be transformed. For that, weight training, which is usually avoided, is the best. With weight lifting, your figure will become more defined, and you'll burn more calories and strengthen your bones. For example, you can run once a week, weight lift once a week, and do something else on the other days. That way, you won't get bored. Company helps fight boredom during exercise. Ask a friend or a neighbor to train with you or join a group. Company makes exercising much more fun and doesn't allow any space for excuses.

12 COMMON MISCONCEPTIONS REGARDING DIET

1. Avoid fat at all costs.

Research has shown that fat has a lot to do with food and drinks that promote weight gain. That doesn't mean that you can consume all kinds of fat. It's very important to track the number of consumed calories and to be aware of your state of health. Increased intake of fats can increase the risk of developing heart disease. Therefore, consume food that contains a low number of saturated fats and fibre, which can be found in whole wheat foods, fruits, and vegetables.

2. Consume dairy products that contain artificially

added calcium.

Some studies show that the body burns more fat if it gets enough calcium. However, we won't get those results if we consume artificially added calcium!

3. We mustn't eat after 6pm.

Cancelling evening meals won't help in achieving results. At most, you will be more tempted to head to the fridge before bed time. Maybe you won't be able to sleep because you'll have to listen to the rumbling in the stomach. Maybe you'll hold yourself away from food to the point that you'll actually eat more than you otherwise would. It's true that it's important what we eat and when we eat it in the evening. It's recommended to eat 3 hours before bed. Yes, we can eat then – but I don't mean the products that have a label "you may".

4. To achieve the desired figure, I have to give up carbohydrates.

Those who decide to eliminate all the carbohydrates in their diet lose weight quite quickly. But, carbohydrates are the main energy source of our body, so a diet like this brings a feeling of fatigue and sleepiness. Of course, some of the carbohydrates (those in bread, pasta, and white rice) are quite fattening, but you can replace them with whole wheat products, fruit, and vegetables.

5. You can eat as much as you want after exercise.

"If I sweat a lot during exercise, I can eat as much as I want after." That belief is not true. Exercise, of course, benefits the physical and mental health (it's proven to help with depression). You must not consume more calories than you burned. Consult a personal trainer or search on the web about how many calories you burn during sport activities. Cycling or long walks burn much fewer calories in comparison to other sports.

6. It is important to withstand in the time of the diet, then you can return to the old ways.

That is also not true, experts say. Those who avoided their favourite foods during the weight-loss time and "cheated" in the end and returned to their old ways didn't achieve any weight progress. Instead of choosing an appropriate diet, you have to change your eating habits. Eat several times, in smaller portions, and write down what you eat and its amount.

7. Skipping meals reduces weight.

This is one of the biggest misconceptions about diet. Skipping meals doesn't reduce weight – all it does is lower the proper functioning of your metabolism and weaken it. Because the body doesn't get enough nutrients because of skipped meals, you will eat more than you normally would the next time you eat.

8. You think you're too young to take care of your health.

There's more and more kids who suffer from diseases connected with obesity – and they only exacerbate with age. Did you know that more and more people develop diabetes and heart diseases in their early twenties? Healthy diet in childhood makes a healthy old age and resistance to diseases.

9. Healthy diet is bland and boring.

Go to a farmer's market or in a well stocked store with

fruits and vegetables and find a taste that suits you the most. Discover food that is tasty and good for your body. Try Mediterranean cuisine, which is healthy, full of flavours, spices, vegetables, and seafood, and is also affordable.

10. Healthy food is expensive.

It is not necessary that healthy food is also expensive. Is salmon on your menu? You can replace it with codfish, a cheaper version of it. Don't buy pre-prepared food. Instead, buy all the ingredients and make the meal yourself. Don't have time for cooking? Prepare casseroles and rolls, pack them, and store them in the fridge or freezer.

11. Usage of so called "low fat" products.

It's right to distinguish between low-fat and low-calorie products. Try to get used to carefully checking the label on a food product, because that is the only way to see how much fat, sugar, and calories it contains. The problem with so called "low fat" products is that our body can produce fat stores from all micro nutrients! These kinds of products often contain large amounts of simple sugars. Often, the product has more calories than its full fat counterpart!

12. Fats are evil and should be avoided.

People think that they will lose weight with a low calorie diet. It's important to know that a third of calories should come from fats, as its necessary for energy, tissue repair, and transportation of vitamins A, D, E, and K around the body.

Focus on ingesting a large amount of fruits and vegetables, which don't have much fat, but contain healthy fibre and vitamins. Unsaturated fats, especially those in walnuts and fish, are especially very healthy.

Some tricks for better success...

Size of Plates and Cutlery

Did you ever think that the size of your plate and cutlery actually effects your meals? Use smaller plates, smaller bowls, high and thin glasses, and smaller spoons. Research has shown that the use of ordinary tablespoons leads to eating 15 percent more food.

High Caloric Drinks

Calories also hide in different flavoured waters and alcoholic beverages. Besides that, we often use carbonated drinks and fruit juices we buy at the store. Even though those drinks contain a lot of calories, they don't satisfy our hunger.

We Drink Too Little Water and Unsweetened Tea

This is one of the most fundamental errors! Before each meal, it's good to drink a glass of liquid. It is even better to have a bottle of water with us at all times, as it ensures that we'll drink more water. Remember that unsweetened liquid is essential for burning calories!

Always Go to the Store with a Shopping List and When You Do Not Feel Hungry.

Before you go to the store, make a shopping list so you don't wander around the shelves. Food on the shelves in stores is arranged very carefully. Many tasty but unneeded products are carefully placed beside the things we need.

If we go to the store feeling hungry, we buy more things than we usually would. Therefore, go to the store after lunch or a snack. You'll save on money and won't buy that many unhealthy foods.

ABOUT THE AUTHOR

Kate Garcia was born in a small city in Europe in a farmers' family. She grew up playing in a backyard, helping family with housekeeping and swimming in nearby river. Later Kate studied agronomy (Bsc) and today she's a business woman running her own business.

She enjoys the warm Spanish weather, endless beaches and most importantly, she has plenty of time to write about her favorites topics. One of them is healthy lifestyle and nutrition. While writing she travels back to her childhood. And she loves it.